I0447434

Painless Dentistry...
It Really Does Happen

The Magic of IV Sedation Dentistry

Laurence E. Fendrich, D.M.D.

Published by:
Laurence E. Fendrich, D.M.D.
Website: www.DentistOnMadison.com

Madison Avenue Dentistry, PLLC
Dental & Sedation Group, LLC

New York City	**Boca Raton/Ft. Lauderdale**
175 Madison Avenue	2028 E. Sample Road
New York, NY 10016	Lighthouse Point, FL 33064

(212) 532-2000

ISBN-13: 978-1480192928
ISBN-10: 1480192929

Painless Dentistry...
It Really Does Happen

The Magic of IV Sedation Dentistry

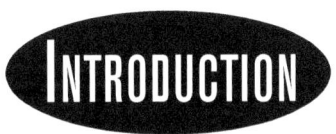

INTRODUCTION

Have you ever been excited about going to the dentist? No? Well, you're not alone. Columbia University's College of Dental Medicine estimates up to fifteen percent of Americans avoid seeing the dentist, due in large part to the anxiety and fear dental visits bring. That's more than forty million people walking around with teeth that are in need – probably *desperate need* – of a professional's attention.

Are you one of them?

Want some more statistics? The US Centers for Disease Control and Prevention reports approximately fifty-three million children and adults have untreated tooth decay. One in three Americans over age thirty has periodontitis, oral advanced gum disease. And nearly three in ten adults over sixty-five have no teeth at all. People tend to think getting dentures when they're older is inevitable, but it's not. It all depends upon how well you take care of your teeth while you've got 'em.

And the first step in doing that is going to your dentist –

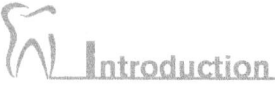

and doing it regularly, not just when emergencies crop up. Most dentists recommend coming in twice a year, unless you're more prone to problems like gum disease (periodontal disease). Then you'd be encouraged to visit more often. Still, that's a problem for some people. Those who are truly *afraid* of going to a dentist's office can't handle even biannual visits. Maybe they had a bad experience once that left them fearful of what might happen if they submit themselves to a dentist again. Maybe their teeth are sensitive, and even routine work can be very painful for them.

On the other hand, some people just don't have *time* to go the dentist. Maybe they're running a business; maybe they travel a lot. They assume – sometimes rightfully so – that they'll go in for a routine exam and X-rays and then be tied to follow-ups for cavities, root canals, or whatever might be found in their initial exam. That could take up valuable time they just don't have to give away.

What we want all these people to know – the phobic ones, the busy ones, and whoever else finds it difficult to deal with going a dentist – is that *there is hope*. They no longer have to put up with painful infections, broken and unsightly teeth, and loose fillings. And instead of going in for appointment after appointment week after week, they can get everything done all at once.

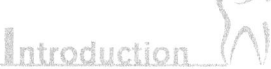

The answer for all of them is **sedation dentistry**.

What does that mean? It's simple. When you have dental work done under sedation, you're given specific medications that will make you unaware of the procedures being performed. You will still be conscious but in a sort of twilight sleep – this isn't like major surgery, where you're anesthetized to the point of being out cold. We practice *conscious sedation*, under which you can respond to stimuli such as the dentist talking to you or an assistant touching your hand, but you won't feel a thing and, most importantly, you will remember little, if anything. Almost any dental procedure can be done under conscious sedation – fillings, implants, root canals, crowns, even routine cleaning and checkups – without worrying about any bad memories of the procedures or any nasty side effects.

Sound good? Well, it is. ***Read on to learn more and find out why sedation dentistry just might be for you.***

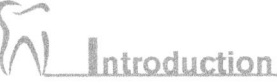

Testimonial

FROM CHRISTIAN S.

When I was a kid, I had an accident and had to have some teeth implants put in. After twenty years or so, my body decided to reject them, and I was left with a problem. Having them replaced would be time-consuming and possibly painful – it was a lot of work that would have to be done probably over many sessions in a dentist's chair.

***That was why I decided to undergo sedation dentistry – so I could get it all done at once without the discomfort of having to listen to all the drilling** and feeling all the pulling of my teeth. Why go through all that anxiety when I didn't have to?*

*I began the process in February 2012 and it was very easy and even relaxing. Under sedation, I felt nothing – no pain whatsoever. The first procedure I had done took only about an hour, **and the results were fantastic. Afterward I went home and took a nap, and that evening I had dinner with my family and watched TV with my kids.** I went back to work the next day.*

***Would I recommend sedation dentistry to others? Absolutely.** There's really no reason to do any sort of oral surgery without it.*

CHAPTER 1

What Is Sedation Dentistry?

Perhaps one of the biggest obstacles people must overcome when it comes to *sedation dentistry* is simply understanding what it is. When you hear that phrase – sedation dentistry – what does it make you think of? Do you imagine yourself lying in a dentist's chair, out cold like you would be if you were having major surgery at a hospital? Or do you think you'll simply pop a pill and go to sleep for a while so the dentist can do the work that needs to be done?

Because there are so many questions floating around about sedation dentistry, and so much misunderstanding, we would like to set the record straight once and for all, starting at the very beginning. The more you know about any medical procedure you will undergo, the more secure you will feel while having it done. So, let's delve into just what it means to have dental work under sedation.

What Is Sedation?

By the simplest definition, *sedation* is a method by which a medical professional administers one or more drugs that will make it easier for a necessary medical procedure to be performed. Specifically, sedation causes the patient to lose consciousness to varying degrees, depending upon what is necessary for the procedure. But equally as important, sedation helps patients by offering these beneficial effects:

- **Anxiolysis**, or a reduction of anxiety and agitation.

- **Amnesia**, or memory lapse for the time during which the sedation is being administered.

- **Analgesia**, or a relief from pain associated with the procedure or the illness or injury it is intended to remedy.

Sedation can be administered through means of inhalation, orally, or intravenously depending upon the procedure being performed and your particular needs as a

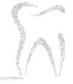

patient. Medications used in sedation generally fall under the categories of benzodiazepines, barbiturates (though these are not too commonly used anymore), non-barbiturate opioids, nonopioids, and inhalation agents.

Okay, now that all the big words are out of the way, let's talk about what sedation *really* means. In a nutshell sedation means total comfort for you! When you have to have any sort of surgery or even a minor procedure done, whether it's in a hospital, a clinic, or a dentist's office, if it involves a level of pain or discomfort that would make the whole thing hard for you to bear – or even make you think twice about having it done at all – then sedation is usually the answer.

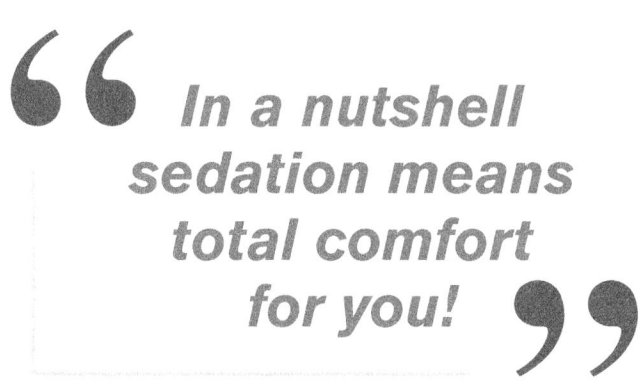

In a nutshell sedation means total comfort for you!

Sedation can make it so you are not aware the procedure is being performed and at the same time reduce your level of pain for the duration. Perhaps most importantly sedation reduces any fear or doubt you might have about the

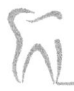

procedure, making it easier for you to have it done – which is especially important when you're faced with something that is necessary for your good health. Often just knowing sedation will be in place reduces a patient's stress and makes him or her more willing even to plan to have a procedure done.

When you're sedated, you feel no pain or discomfort; often you feel nothing at all and remember little if anything of the procedure, depending on which methods and medications are employed. Doesn't that sound good? Imagine having to go in for some work – oral surgery, dental implants, some dental crowns, or anything you feel a little queasy about doing – and being sedated, then waking up later with the work done, the pain gone, and no nasty memories of any of it in your mind. This is one of the great appeals of sedation dentistry to some people – there are no anxiety-inducing flashbacks to worry about. But we'll get into such perks a little bit later.

Where Did It Come From?

Even though we administer sedation on a daily basis, we still sometimes wonder: who on earth thought up such a thing? It's like the old question about the crazy guy who decided to milk a cow for the first time – and then drank what he got out of it. What kind of mad genius comes up with ideas like this?

Well, in a word: **a dentist**. That's right, the inventor of what we now know as sedation was a dentist. William T.G. Morton of Massachusetts first worked as a clerk, a printer, and a salesman before enrolling in the Baltimore College of Dentistry in 1840. Two years later he left the school to join a dental partnership in Connecticut, then two years after that entered Harvard Medical School (at the behest of his fiancée's parents, who for some reason objected to the dental profession).

At Harvard, William learned about ether, an anesthetic, and began to see its potential as a sedation medicine. On September 30, 1846, he put his theory to the test and administered ether to a patient undergoing a tooth extraction — and it worked. The patient felt no pain. To say this was a breakthrough in a world where dental work could be a brutal undertaking is an understatement.

Morton's phenomenal feat was covered in a newspaper in Boston, where the procedure took place. The article caught the eye of local surgeon Henry Bigelow, who then demonstrated the same technique during a surgery to remove a tumor. Again the procedure was completed and the patient felt no pain. William T.G. Morton's discovery was a bone fide success — and the practice we know today as *sedation* became legitimate medicine.

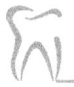

All thanks to a dentist!

The <u>Four</u> Levels of Sedation

When we say *sedation* most people think of what it's like when they have some sort of major surgery. They believe they will be totally unconscious, unable to respond to any stimuli as their medical procedure is performed.

Sometimes that is the case. However it's not like that all the time. In fact there are four different levels of sedation, ranging from just making you a little drowsy to full-on knocking you out. Which one you need depends upon a myriad of factors such as your personal medical history and the type of procedure you're having done.

Let's take a look at each of them up close.

1. Minimal Sedation

Also known as *anxiolysis*. Under minimal sedation you respond to verbal instructions pretty much as you normally would when not sedated. Your breathing and heart functioning remain normal. The main purpose of minimal sedation is to make you less nervous, not to put you completely out of commission. In dentistry, nitrous oxide (laughing gas) is used for this.

2. Moderate (Conscious) Sedation

Sometimes also called *conscious sedation*. Under moderate sedation you can still respond to verbal commands and/or tactile cues. Moderate sedation causes a depression of your consciousness – but you can still breathe on your own and your heart function will remain normal. In dental and medical procedures, we call this IV conscious (or moderate) sedation.

3. Deep Sedation

Under deep sedation you are asleep and cannot be easily woken, and you will only respond to stimulation that is repeated or painful. Your ability to breathe on your own might be impaired, but your heart should function as normal.

4. General Anesthesia

With this method you fully lose consciousness. You cannot be woken by verbal, tactile, or even painful stimulation. You will need assistance breathing (via a ventilator) and your heart function might become impaired as well.

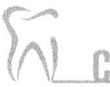

Generally speaking if you need highly invasive or complex surgery, you're looking at number four – you will need to be fully unconscious simply because of the length of the procedure and the pain level involved. For someone who has minimal fear of dentistry or needles, something like number one might be adequate before performing noninvasive dental work; using laughing gas and Novocain or lidocaine.

In our sedation dentistry practice, we utilize number two: moderate or IV conscious sedation. We like this option because it offers us greater, tighter control over the medications you receive and how they affect you. It also has less side effects than heavier methods while giving you enough sedation to ensure your experience will be pleasant. Of course we will go into much more detail about this a little bit later.

Sedation Dentistry: How It Works

If you're considering having some dental work done while under sedation, you probably have a lot of questions floating around in your head: What on earth are they going to do to me? How is this sedation going to happen? Will I have to take pills? Will needles be involved?

And the answers to these questions depend on what sort of work you're having done and on where and by whom you're having it done. Customs, preferences, and even regulations differ from practice to practice and from state to state, so depending on your particular circumstance, you might wind up with any of these <u>three</u> traditional methods:

1. Nitrous Oxide

Or, as it's more commonly known, laughing gas. This is a colorless gas with a slightly sweet odor and taste that can suppress pain but not knock you out; with laughing gas you're conscious and aware and can carry on regular conversations. It's been used in dentistry since 1863 and is the most widely used gas anesthetic in dentistry today.

2. Oral Sedation

This means pills – the kind that take away some of the anxiety you might feel and help you to relax. The most common anti-anxiety pills used in dentistry are benzodiazepenes; some brand names you might recognize include Valium, Halcion, Xanax, and Ativan. Generally you would take one of these pills the night before your appointment and then another about an hour before you arrive at your dentist's office. They will not knock you out, but they will make you more calm and relaxed. Hey, they don't call them *happy pills* for nothing.

3. IV Sedation

This is when the sedation agent – usually in the form of benzodiazepenes and/or opioids – is administered directly into your body in liquid form. It's just like you would have if you were in a hospital for any reason.

> " *In our opinion IV sedation is the most effective method when it comes to keeping a patient safe and comfortable during dental work...* "

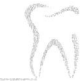

> **" Who wants to sit in a chair, staring up at a light, waiting for a pill to kick in while their mind races with nightmares about what the procedure is going to entail? "**

In our opinion IV sedation is the most effective method when it comes to keeping a patient safe and comfortable during dental work – and it's what we use at our office. Administering sedative agents through an IV quickly brings a patient into a relaxed state, which is so important for someone who suffers from any type of dental phobia. Who wants to sit in a chair, staring up at a light, waiting for a pill to kick in while their mind races with nightmares about what the procedure is going to entail?

With IV sedation this waiting period is negligible, and a patient's anxiety can be alleviated simply, rapidly, and safely. More importantly IV sedation allows closer control and monitoring of a patient's level of sedation throughout a procedure. Getting too relaxed? Ease up on the medication. Starting to feel something? Add in a little bit more medication. It all depends on what works best for you – and with IV sedation, we can monitor that from moment to moment. *(See the "What to Expect" section of this book for further details about exactly how IV sedation is administered.)*

A Closer Look at Medications

Benzodiazepenes, opioids – they sound impressive, but what on earth are they? Let's take a look at them a little more in depth so you can become more familiar with the drugs you might be required to take if you choose to have· sedation dentistry.

Benzodiazepenes, or *benzos* for short, work specifically to reduce anxiety and bring on sedation. They do this by affecting the brain: some benzos target areas that control emotions such as fear and anxiety while others work on the parts of your brain that regulate sleeping and wakefulness. Generally benzodiazepenes in lower doses reduce anxiety; at higher levels they bring on sedation. In either case they depress the central nervous system, which causes a slight decline in blood pressure and respiration – but not drastically so. Just enough to keep you from feeling too anxious.

Opioids are painkillers that are generally used in conjunction with benzodiazepenes when a stronger analgesic or sedative effect is required. Opioids work by binding to receptors in the central nervous system and gastrointestinal tract and through them decreasing the patient's perception of pain; sedation is merely a side effect of this. Examples of commonly used opioids you might recognize include morphine, fentanyl, and Demerol.

What Do the Experts Say?

In 2000, the American Association of Oral and Maxillofacial Surgeons (AAOMS) conducted a study to determine the effects of anesthesia (local and general) and sedation (conscious and deep) on patients undergoing dental and oral surgery. The study included 34,191 patients who had work done at 79 different dental practices – making it the largest study of its kind. Of those patients 71.9 percent underwent deep sedation and general anesthesia, 15.5 percent had conscious sedation, and 12.6 percent received local anesthesia.

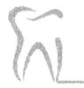

The result? In a nutshell sedation dentistry is extremely safe and very well received by patients who undergo it.

> " *... Sedation dentistry is extremely safe and very well received by patients who undergo it.* "

But let's look at the results in greater detail:

- In the study there were 1.3 complications in every 100 cases — all of which were minor. Only 2 patients out of the 34,191 involved required hospitalization.

- Over 80 percent of the patients in the study reported feeling anxious before their procedures;

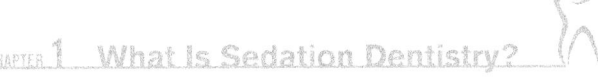

afterward over 61 percent said they would not fear having similar procedures done in the future. Obviously they enjoyed the experience!

- Overall 94.3 percent of those involved in the study were satisfied with the anesthetic treatment they received (which included sedation).

- More than 94 percent of them said they would recommend the same methods to their loved ones.

Numbers like that – they speak for themselves.

Our Qualifications

Whenever you see a doctor for any sort of treatment, you want to make sure he or she has the proper credentials and training to give you the level of service and care you need. This goes double for a practitioner of IV sedation dentistry. There are so many factors that go into sedation, from knowing the right medications to use to experience in monitoring a sedate patient to any number of other incidentals that might crop up while the procedure is being performed. You simply have to ensure the dentist you're seeing knows what he or she is doing.

In our practice we are fully trained and licensed in the area of IV conscious sedation dentistry and have completed – and often go above and beyond – the demanding requirements of the state of Florida:

■ We have performed more than 11,000 IV sedations in our practice with *not one* significant medical complication.

■ We have attended rigorous post-graduate courses in dental anesthesia.

■ We have continuous training in advanced cardiac life support.

Most states require dentists who administer anesthesia to be trained only in basic cardiac life support, which is the basic CPR class anyone can take. But in the interest of the safety of our patients, we have surpassed that and instead are accomplished in *advanced* cardiac life support (ACLS). Instead of just learning how to resuscitate someone (which is very important), we have been trained in performing, reading, and interpreting EKGs, managing airway problems, and solving acute medical emergencies, all so we can monitor and respond to changes in our patients' heart rhythms while they are under sedation. For further monitoring we use blood pressure cuffs and pulse oximeters – the clip that goes on

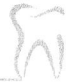

your fingertip to monitor your blood's oxygen saturation level — to keep a second-by-second watch on our patients' vital signs.

Basically whatever we can do to ensure our patients are comfortable, stable, and stress-free is what we do. Whether it falls under the basic requirements we must meet as doctors or takes us a step or three above, we will do it. To us nothing is more important than your safety.

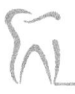
Testimonial

FROM DAVID T.

I decided to have my dental work done under sedation because it was such a large job – and because, I'll admit, I've always had a big fear of dentists. Once, when I was a kid, I'd had some work done and wasn't given enough Novocain, and I've never forgotten that experience. Sedation, I figured, could calm my nerves and allow the dentist to do what needed to be done all in one shot.

At my consultation I found out I had several top teeth that needed to be extracted and would need four implants placed as well. I would also be fitted for a new bottom denture as the one I had no longer fit me correctly. When you're talking about extracting ten or fifteen teeth and grinding down bone – well, no one would want to be awake to feel all that pressure and pulling and yanking. Sedation dentistry was the only way to go.

Everything about the experience I had was great. The people at the office were very cordial; they even arranged rides to and from the facility for me and made sure I got in my house safely after my work was done. They went over very clearly what they needed to do for the procedure so I understood what would happen. Dr. Fendrich gave me many options to choose from when it came to working on my uppers and did what he

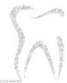
Testimonial

FROM DAVID T.

CONTINUED ● ● ● ● ● ● ● ● ● ● ● ●▶

could to work within my budget. I have to say too that he's not afraid to tackle the difficult jobs – I'd had quadruple bypass a year earlier and was on blood thinners at the time of the dental work, and he and his staff were able to do all my work under sedation despite that.

We scheduled two separate appointments: one to place the three lower implants and do some bone restructuring in my jaw, and one to do the top extractions. Once I was under sedation, for both procedures, everything went perfectly. The first session took three and a half to four hours, and the second lasted four or five hours. Not once in all that time did I feel any pain – I didn't even feel the shots of Novocain I had to get.

Afterward I was sleepy, which is normal. Once I got home I slept for the rest of the day, getting up one or twice as I needed to. Other than that I had no lingering side effects from the sedation.

I would absolutely recommend sedation dentistry to anyone who has a lot of work to be done.

Testimonial

FROM LAURIE Q.

I am the most bizarre patient. I have very sensitive teeth, and getting any sort of work done on them is always very painful. It's very difficult for anyone to touch them, and I've been to dentists who actually refused even to clean my teeth because of it.

So, I looked into sedation dentistry. I found Dr. Fendrich on the Internet, and his practice had such good reviews, I called right away to make an appointment. When I went in for a consultation, everyone was so nice and friendly, I decided to give it a shot and have some work done there. I ended up needing porcelain crowns on all my top teeth.

I ended up having two sedations done, each appointment, from arrival to departure, lasting about five hours. And I didn't feel a thing. I was never in any pain. Afterward I went home and slept, and the next day I was back at work. I highly recommend sedation dentistry to everyone. It was the best for me.

CHAPTER 2

Who Should Undergo Sedation Dentistry?

That's easy: *almost anyone.*

No, really. Almost anyone can utilize conscious (IV conscious sedation) during dental work, and everyone can find some benefit in it – as long as you're over fifteen years old and in good health, though even if you're not in good health, we can usually work something out. We'd love so much for everyone to give it a try, we do everything we can to make it accessible.

However, there are certain people sedation dentistry can help the most.

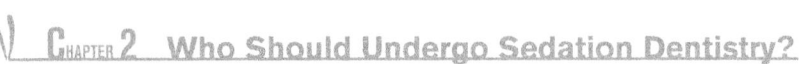

People With Phobias

Fear comes in all shapes and sizes. Some of us don't like heights. Others go all cold when they see a spider. People have phobias about everything from airplanes to clowns to the number thirteen. (Really – it's called triskaidekaphobia.) Some of these may seem silly, but to a person suffering from the phobia, it's no joke. A phobia can be a truly painful experience and can severely limit one's life.

Perhaps the worst are the medical phobias. This includes the fear of needles (trypanophobia), hospitals (nosocomephobia), medical procedures (tomophobia), medications (pharmacophobia), even doctors and dentists (Iatrophobia) themselves. Sometimes medical phobias are referred to as *white-coat syndrome* because of the white coats medical professionals tend to wear – with the assumption that just seeing one will cause some people anxiety.

Medical phobias, and dental phobia in particular, might not affect a person's everyday life, but in the long run they can be quite detrimental. Consider this: You have a mild toothache, but fear keeps you from going to see a dentist. The toothache gets worse and worse, going from a mild ache and sensitivity to sharp, ongoing pain. Untreated, this can lead to serious infection that can spread throughout your body.

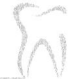

If this sounds like you, sedation dentistry can be the key to maintaining good oral health. Sedation allows a dentist to perform whatever procedures need to be done, from deep cleaning to crowns, while allowing you to enjoy an easy, stress-free experience. Yes, *enjoy*. With sedation dentistry, no matter how difficult your phobia may be, it will be possible for you to have a positive visit to the dentist.

> *... Sedation dentistry can be the key to maintaining good oral health.*

Very Busy People

I know what you're thinking: how busy do you really have to be not to be able to make it to several dentist appointments? In this day and age, you might be surprised. People who work a

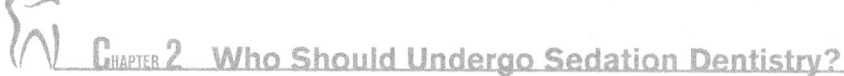
lot, parents of young children, even those with very active social calendars can sometimes find it challenging to go to multiple dental visits and take care of themselves as well as they should.

As noted in the introduction, up to fifteen percent of Americans are overdue for a visit to the dentist, yet continue to avoid it. The problem is, many of them cannot help it. They know they have lots of dental problems but don't go, then blame it on time constraints and this busy world we live in.

For people like this, again, sedation dentistry can be the answer. Instead of coming in for a visit for deep cleaning, then again the following week for fillings, then the following week for a root canal and crown, under IV sedation all this can be taken care of in one simple, restful visit. Normally a dentist wouldn't consent to do so many procedures in one sitting for a few different reasons, but time is the biggest factor – most people would get antsy and uncomfortable if they had to sit in a dentist's chair for as long as it would take to do everything.

IV Sedation dentistry avoids this by making it so the patient doesn't even realize how much time has passed. While sedated, you are unaware of your surroundings and any discomfort. With the patient in this relaxed state, the dentist can more easily and effectively perform all the work that needs to be done in one visit, eliminating the need for future visits. In many cases, when you wake up from the sedation, you can simply get back to your busy lifestyle and not worry about having to make time to see the dentist again. At least not for another six months.

People With Complex Dental Issues

With so many people not visiting their dentists on a regular basis, it's no surprise many of them end up with complex dental issues. This means not just your run-of-the-mill cavities and plaque but things like root canals, extractions, dental restorations or implants, crowns, or a combination of all of the above and/or other issues.

When a situation like this arises, often people are put off from going to the dentist because they fear the pain they might have to endure or even the judgment of the dental professionals in the office. (And if you feel your dentist is judging you, let us give you a tip: drop him/her and get a new one. He/she should be there to help you, not to make you feel worse than you already do.)

With sedation dentistry, however, there's no need to fear seeking the attention you need, no matter what kind of shape your mouth is in. Even people with the worst cases of gum disease, tooth decay, or a host of other problems can undergo dental procedures with the help of sedation and come out feeling good about themselves and feeling healthier because they've had all their dental problems fixed.

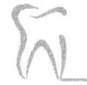

> " *Even people with the worst cases of gum disease, tooth decay, or a host of other problems can undergo dental procedures with the help of sedation and come out feeling good and healthier about themselves because they've had all their dental problems fixed.* "

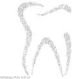

The Benefits of Sedation Dentistry

We could go on and on about the types of people who can find benefits in the use of sedation dentistry, but that would make quite a long book. These have been just a few examples of issues people have found relief for through sedation dentistry. Whether your issues are encompassed by the information here or are something completely unique, no doubt you too can be helped by sedation dentistry. All you have to do is be willing to give it a try.

And if you do, what exactly will be in store for you? Well, we'll look in depth at the actual sedation dentistry process in the next chapter. But right now, let's look at its benefits. As you can imagine, sedation dentistry has many of the same benefits as dental work performed on a conscious patient: better oral health, avoidance of future related health issues throughout the body, and of course all the positive aesthetic aspects of having a gleaming, beautiful smile.

But on top of all that, sedation dentistry has some *bonus* advantages. First and foremost, there will be no pain. While under sedation, you will not feel the needles, the drills, or any of the hurt that can be associated with dental procedures. Second, you'll have no recollection of the work. That means no flashbacks or nightmares, just the end result – your perfect teeth – with none of the heartache.

> **"** *While under sedation, you will not feel the needles, the drills, or any of the hurt that can be associated with dental procedures.* **"**

As we've already mentioned, if you're a busy guy or gal, sedation dentistry allows you to get a lot of work done in a little bit of time, and that, to some, is one of its biggest benefits.

Whatever your reasons for looking into sedation dentistry, you'll undoubtedly find something about it that appeals to you. Everyone's dental experiences are unique – as individual to us as our teeth themselves. But there is one thing we all have in common: no matter who we are or what we need to have done, we can all benefit from sedation dentistry. Some of us just don't know it yet!

Testimonial

FROM LEE L.

I'm not a fan of having anyone work on my mouth. I don't like anyone touching it. That's why I sought out sedation dentistry. And I knew Dr. Fendrich was the right dentist because he's such a warm person; he really makes his patients feel like part of the family.

At my consultation I found out I had one tooth that was rotted below the gum line – the root was rotted and infected underneath the crown. I was on vacation at the time and was not happy about the pain it caused. Dr. Fendrich took full X-rays and showed me all the problems I had – many of which I had brought to the attention of other dentists, and they'd told me there was nothing wrong. If I'd listened to them, I would have lost my teeth.

I went home and discussed my options with my husband, and we decided to go with sedation dentistry. I had two implants put in and I don't know how many crowns, but everything was done in one day – the entire appointment took four hours. Later, when I'm fully healed, I will go back to have teeth put in

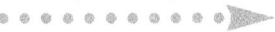

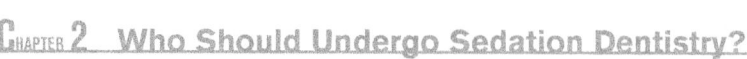

Testimonial

FROM LEE L.

CONTINUED ● ● ● ● ● ● ● ● ● ● ● ◗

where the implants are now. After that I'll continue with some other work I need done in the front.

When I had my dental work done under sedation, I felt no pain at all, and I woke up with a smile. *I had no reaction to the sedation, no sickness, and I'd felt no pain during the procedure. I'd never had an experience like it in my life. I went home and laid down and rested for a while – mostly because my husband wanted me to, not because I really felt like I needed to. Then I called up my old dentist and told him I was never going back to his practice. I live in Georgia, and I'm not rich – it's not like I can just take a plane down to Florida anytime I want to see Dr. Fendrich. But when I have to, I will. He's worth it to me. He really makes his patients feel like part of the family.*

I would definitely recommend sedation dentistry to other people – really, I don't see any other way.

FROM LYNN G.

I hate going to the dentist. I had a bad experience with one – all he wanted to do was max my insurance out. He kept calling me and trying to talk me into having more work done, and I got sick of it.

But then my cheek swelled up, and I knew I needed dental help. I'd heard of Dr. Fendrich's practice and knew they did sedation, so I figured I'd go that route. After a consultation he agreed. The work I had to get done – extraction of the broken, infected molar that had caused the swelling, an implant, and crowns on two teeth on the top right – would be painful. I wanted to be asleep for it.

The experience of sedation was great. I don't remember anything – only speaking with Dr. Fendrich that morning when he came in to say hello. The entire appointment took about three hours, and when the procedure was done I had no lingering pain. I went home and slept until around 6:30 that evening, got up and had a little to eat, then went back to sleep. But that's to be expected – and it was a good sleep!

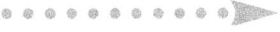

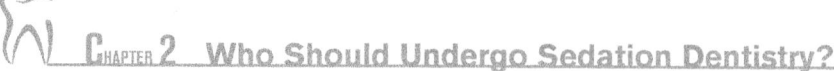

Testimonial

FROM LYNN G.

CONTINUED ● ● ● ● ● ● ● ● ● ● ● ➤

I went back the following day for a checkup. My mouth had swelled a bit, but Dr. Fendrich explained to me that he'd had to reconstruct some bone in the area where he was working – the work had been extensive. He told me I'd have swelling for a few days, and every day it went down more.

I would absolutely recommend sedation dentistry, especially when you're having extensive stuff done, like I did. Overall Dr. Fendrich's office is immaculate, and the staff is very nice, professional, and caring. They have followed up with me every step of the way to see how I'm feeling. Dr. Fendrich is nice too, and a straight shooter, which I appreciate.

CHAPTER 3

What to Expect

So you've made the decision: sedation dentistry is for you. Or, at least, you think it is. If you like what you've read so far and think having dental work performed under IV conscious sedation sounds good, the next step you should take is scheduling an appointment so you and your dentist can determine *together* what you need to have done. Then you can talk about sedation and whether or not it will work out best for you.

 **So you've made the decision: sedation dentistry is for you.**

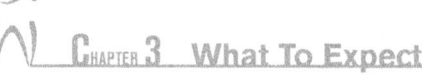

And after that? Well, like everything else in life, having dental work done is a process – and conscious sedation is just another thing that gets added to the process. However, don't worry; it's an easy one. From the first moment of your consultation through the completion of your work done under IV conscious sedation, your experience will be a stress-free one. After all, that's the whole point of sedation dentistry: to keep you in good health with as little hassle as possible.

Your Initial Visit

Sedation dentistry is not the same at every practice; routines, procedures, and even laws differ from one dentist to another and from state to state. So, we can't guarantee here what you might find if you go into your local dentist and ask to have work done under IV conscious sedation. But we can tell you what you can expect if you come to our practice.

When you first come in, you will be treated with respect. No matter how much or how little you need to have done, no matter what sort of shape your teeth and mouth are in, we want to help you. We want to take care of you. And we want to do it in a way that works best for you.

For many people, this will indeed mean undergoing dental work using IV conscious sedation. For others sedation

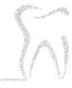

will not be necessary. How do you know which method will be best for you? That's something we'll help you decide during your consultation.

First we'll do some X-rays of your mouth in order to assess what dental procedures you might need to have done. We'll look at them together so you can see where your problem areas lie. Then we'll talk about your comfort level with that list of tasks. If you feel good about being in a dentist's office and comfortable with the work you'll have done (especially if it might include needles), then we'll most likely recommend just jumping right into it. While sedation is extremely safe – especially when performed at our practice; as mentioned earlier, we truly go above and beyond the call of duty when it comes to training and precautions – not everyone needs it. If you have no problem with having dental work done, then chances are IV conscious sedation will not be necessary for you. All you need is a regular appointment.

For those who are hesitant or who feel uncomfortable just being in a dentist's office, sedation will undoubtedly be a topic of discussion during the consultation. We'll tell you how it's done, how it will make you feel, and both the benefits and potential drawbacks of pursuing this course (and there are very few drawbacks!). If and when you decide to go with sedation, we'll set up an appointment for you at a later time, have you sign some routine consent forms, and give you a few

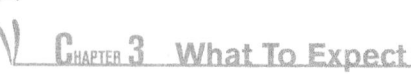

prescriptions to prepare you for the procedure. It's as simple as that, and you're on your way to better dental health.

The night before your appointment, we'll ask you to take one of the prescriptions we gave you: either Xanax or Triazolam (also known as Halcion), a sedative just to take the edge off. This will help you sleep well and ensure you're not up all night worrying about the procedures you have scheduled for the next day. The next day you'll take one more pill, one hour before your appointment. This second dose will allow us to give you less of the stronger medications once you get to the office.

In many other dental practices, this is where the medication ends; if the pills begin to wear off, you simply have to take another, then maybe another. Though we understand this is all some practices are licensed to do, or sometimes even all that is allowed by law, we believe it's unsafe. Say a big linebacker of a man is given one Halcion, then two, then three, and he's still not feeling sleepy enough to have his dental work done. If he's pushed to a fourth dose, who knows what will happen? Maybe that medication has built up in his bloodstream and the rapid addition of just one more pill will cause his blood pressure to crash. He could end up hospitalized just from trying to get some dental work done – and not even get the work done at all.

With IV conscious sedation, we can tightly monitor your dosages and keep them at therapeutic levels that will in no way harm you. If you're not sleepy enough, we can give you a little more; if you seem too sedated, we'll pull back right away. This is the beauty of it – every aspect is completely in control. We also keep a close watch on your vital signs, including pulse, heart function, and blood pressure. If any fluctuations occur we can address them right away, change the medication dosages if necessary, and avoid any serious problems.

With IV conscious sedation, we can tightly monitor your dosages and keep them at therapeutic levels that will in no way harm you.

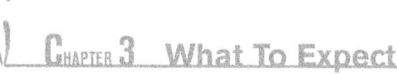
Back to the day of your appointment. After you've taken your second dose of Xanax or Triazolam, you may be concerned about driving to our office — but don't be. As part of our outstanding service, we have a transportation aide come to pick you up and drive you in — yes, you get your own concierge. This is just another way we try to take the pressure off of you so you can focus on relaxing and getting your work done — and maybe even enjoying the experience in the process.

When you reach our office, one of our fantastic staff members will greet you. By this point, thanks to the medication, you'll be starting to feel pretty relaxed. Some people are able to walk just fine while others may need a little help. One of our assistants will bring you to a room that's already been set up for you and help you get settled in one of our really comfortable dental chairs. They will recline you, help you to relax further, and then sit with you and review your medical history — standard procedure just to make sure everything's in order before we administer any medications to you. They'll also review what work you'll have done at the appointment, and one of us — the dentists — will come in to talk to you as well.

When all these formalities are done, the assistant will take your initial vital signs, including your blood pressure and heart rate. Then you'll be hooked up to an EKG to get a baseline of your heart activity. This is so that during the procedure, we will know what's normal for you – and be able to react right away if we see that any of these vital signs change. If no issues are found in our initial assessment, we'll get started with your IV sedation and then your dental care. *Remember:* our method of doing IV sedation is extremely safe and we always want you to be as healthy as possible before you undergo it so that it will be a stress-free, enjoyable, and – above all – safe experience.

Once we start your intravenous line, we'll begin to administer some medications that will gradually make you more and more restful. We don't have a standard amount of medications that we give to all people. Since all people are different – some have blond hair or brown, some are tall or short – the medication levels they require are usually a little different as well. Some people may need a minimal amount to get sleepy while others may need more. The doses you receive are based on your body's makeup including your height and weight, your past and current medical conditions, and how robust we feel your system seems to be. We use a method of administering medications called *titration*, in which we keep adding very small doses of medication until we get you to the desired state of sedation. *We judge this by evaluating you and asking ourselves a few questions:*

- ◼ Can you respond when we speak to you or touch you on the shoulder?

- ◼ What are your vital signs? How do they compare to the baseline we took on you when you arrived for your appointment?

- ◼ Can you clear your lungs by yourself? Is your breathing regular?

If the answer to any of these questions is "no," then there might be a problem and we will immediately pull back on the IV sedation. None of the medications we give are permanent or long-lasting; if you need to wake up immediately we can administer another drug to counteract anything we've already given you. The drugs we use are completely reversible. We can bring you back to full consciousness in less than fifteen seconds if we have to.

Eventually, as the medication does its work, you will become very sleepy, and that's the point at which we know we can start your dental care. You won't be unconscious; you'll still be breathing on your own and have spontaneous heart activity. You'll still be able to respond when someone talks to

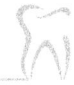

you – you just won't feel anything being done in your mouth. We will also administer pain medication throughout your procedure – something like... fentanyl for short procedures, Demerol for slightly longer procedures, and morphine if you really need a lot of work done.

When your dental work is complete, we'll stop your IV and give you those counteracting medications to bring you out of your conscious sedation. It won't take you long to become alert, but we'll give you time to rest as well, to be sure you're physically ready to leave. Before you do, we will again sit down and go over the procedure with you, letting you know how everything went. We'll give you after-care instructions – in writing – that you'll need to follow for a few days and go over them with you as well, point by point, just to be sure you understand them. Since you still might be groggy, you will not be required to sign anything at this point; you already took care of that at your initial consultation. Now you just have to think about taking care of yourself – and how good your mouth will soon be feeling.

When you're well enough to get up and walk, we'll escort you outside again, where your transportation aide will be waiting to drive you home. Once there you'll most likely want to lie down and sleep for a few hours. There are no lasting side effects of IV conscious sedation, but the medications can take up to twelve hours to leave your body, so you'll be tired

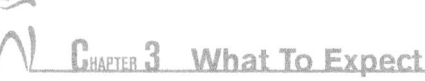

for a while. It's a good idea to take the day off from work and not make any plans if you're going to have dental work done under conscious sedation.

The best part of this whole experience will come when you wake up from your nap and get up to look at yourself in your bathroom mirror. Open wide, and we're sure you're going to like what you see. Whatever problems your teeth had will be gone, a beaming, beautiful smile in their place. And even better, you'll have no memory of what it took to get it that way.

FROM **LYNN J.**

Like many other people, I had a bad experience with a dentist, and now I don't like them. When I needed work done, it took me six months to research online and find Dr. Fendrich. When I contacted his office, the staff was so nice to me. I felt comfortable... but then I got nervous, and I cancelled my appointment. A couple of weeks later I rescheduled. I'm a very nervous person.

All in all I had twenty dental implants placed — ten on the bottom and ten on top. And I didn't feel anything through the procedure. I didn't even know there were needles involved, and I have no scars. The sedation had no side effects, not even a headache. When I felt sleepy and I rested — that was about it.

Over time I've had five separate sedation dentistry sessions. The first one lasted five hours, the second another five; I put in three and a half hours in February and then another hour and a half to finish up.

I would recommend sedation dentistry to anyone who is nervous like I am. The girls who work in Dr. Fendrich's office are like saints. They held my hand and everything. I've already had my husband go there for a crown, and I'm trying to convince my brother-in-law to go too.

Testimonial

FROM STEPHANIE H.

I needed major work done. I'd had sedation dentistry done before, by another dentist. He have me an Ativan or Xanax to relax me, and that was for major, five to six hour surgery.

I had heard about Dr. Fendrich, so I called him as a second consultant, to give me his opinion on how I should proceed. and what procedures to have done? With him I had two teeth pulled and three implants placed in my lower jaw. When they're done healing I'll go back to have my crowns redone, fix an old bridge that's decaying underneath, and have some teeth removed. Whereas the first dentist I saw had said he would leave whatever work he did in my mouth open to heal, Dr. Fendrich made a very nice temporary bridge to go over the implants, so it looks like I have normal teeth.

I had no problems at all with the procedure – no pain or anything. It took about five and a half hours – Dr. Fendrich

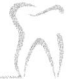

FROM **STEPHANIE H.**

CONTINUED

and his team ended up pulling two teeth and placing three implants. This involved my whole lower right jaw. They also repaired my crowns on the other side. I especially liked that they had someone to pick me up before the procedure and drive me home when it was done.

Afterward I had no side effects. There was discomfort, but Dr. Fendrich gave me medication to get me through – just over the counter Advil. Nothing unusual. I was tired because of the sedation, so I went home, put ice on my mouth, and slept for eight to ten hours off and on.

I would absolutely recommend sedation dentistry, and particularly Dr. Fendrich. He's very nice – his whole staff is.

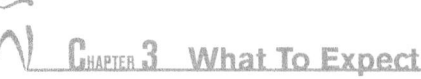

FROM **SANDRA C.**

I'm seventy-three years old, and sedation dentistry appealed to me. Not just because of my age but because I have a son with traumatic brain injury, and I can't be away from him long. Sedation offered the speed I needed and the lack of pain I wanted. I had all my teeth capped years ago and have a lot of history with dentists, and I just didn't want to go through the same thing again.

In all I had eight implants done under sedation, and it went perfectly. Afterward I felt a little groggy and sleepy, but that was it. I would absolutely, incontrovertibly recommend it, especially people who need extensive work done but are afraid.

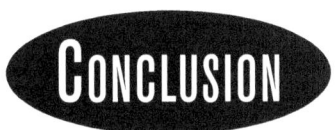

CONCLUSION

There is hope.

This is the message we want you to take from this book. We've said it from the beginning, and we'll repeat it right up to the end: no matter how bad your dental phobia is, no matter how much you hate needles, no matter how much work you need done, there is hope. You can have good dental health. And you *can* have it on your own terms.

People who undergo IV conscious sedation dentistry come from all walks of life, and they use sedation for a variety of reasons. Some have true dental phobias that inhibit them from having work done in their mouths. Maybe their anxiety comes from a bad past experience; maybe it's something they just can't explain. Some people have extremely sensitive teeth, making even routine checkups uncomfortable or painful. Others are always on the go – they simply don't have time in their schedules for the repeated visits it would take to get everything done.

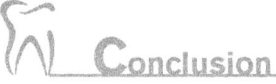

Whatever _your_ reason is, we can work with it. There is hope, and no matter your issue, your dental work can get done.

Many people, when they hear about sedation dentistry, imagine being hospitalized and put under general anesthesia, as if they were undergoing major surgery. But it's nothing like that. Sedation dentistry utilizes what's called conscious or IV sedation, which simply makes you unaware of the procedure being performed, but you are not "knocked out." You feel like you're asleep, but you can still respond to questions and directions. You breathe on your own, and your heart function remains normal. Best of all, your level of pain for the duration of the work is zero – as is any fear or doubt you might have about getting it done.

Ask any of our patients who've had it done. Or better yet, go back and reread the "**Testimonials**" throughout this book. You can hear it in their own words:

▶ _"It was the best decision I ever made."_

▶ _"I felt no pain at all, and I woke up with a smile."_

▶ _"It went perfectly."_

▶ _"I would absolutely recommend sedation dentistry."_

That's a word we hear a lot: *absolutely*. Once people undergo IV conscious sedation dentistry to have their dental work done, they can't wait to tell people about it – and to absolutely recommend they try it themselves. Those are the kinds of positive experiences we strive to create. That is how we give people hope.

How else do we inspire our patients?

- **Simply by being the best at what we do.**
  Our doctors and all staff involved in our procedures are fully trained and licensed in IV conscious sedation dentistry and have completed – and often go above and beyond – the demanding requirements of the state of Florida.

- **By backing it up with numbers.**
  To date we have performed more than 11,000 IV sedations in our practice with not one significant medical complication.

- **By going the extra mile.**
  We'll not only arrange to have you picked up and dropped off at home on the day of your procedure; we'll hold your hand through the whole thing if that's what you need. We're here for you, to give

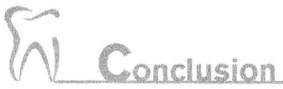
you the help that you need — whatever form that might come in.

■ By working with your schedule.
Have kids who keep you running from morning till night? A demanding job? Travel a lot? No problem. We can fit you in. One of the advantages of sedation dentistry is that you can get a lot of work out of the way in a short time. We'll help you maximize your time by getting in, getting it done, and getting on with your life.

■ By explaining everything.
From your initial consultation to your after-care follow-up appointment, we will keep you in the loop on your own dental health. So many people feel afraid of dentists simply because they don't understand what's going on or why they need a particular procedure performed. That's not how we "operate." We want you to participate in your care, not be just a bystander. The more you know, the more you confident you'll feel, and the more willing you'll be to get the work done.

FROM **WAYNE S.**

I've had bad experiences with dentists in the past – real horror stories. When I was younger a tooth cracked on my upper jaw, and I had to have root canal done. That was when I discovered how little Novocain worked on me. When my wisdom teeth were pulled, I tried nitrous oxide, but I felt everything that was going on. I heard the crunching and felt the pain.

Under sedation I ended up having all of my upper teeth replaced with caps. The sedation worked great. I didn't feel pain at all. Normally, when Novocain and nitrous oxide didn't work for me, I would have to take a lot of painkillers afterward. With sedation I took none. I had three procedures done, one for four hours and the other two for two hours each, and after each one I was just tired. That's the only side effect. I would recommend sedation dentistry to anyone.

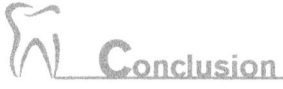

Testimonial

FROM ALICIA W.

Having my dental work done under sedation was the best decision I ever made. I needed lots of teeth removed – my lowers were very bad and nine of them needed to come out at one time. Many years ago I had general anesthesia and that didn't go well for me. Under sedation I could respond to commands and cooperate; there was no breathing tube, so no sore throat, and I didn't feel hungover when it was time to wake up.

The sedation was minimal. I felt just two little pricks when the IVs were placed at my elbow and on back of my hand, and I didn't even bruise from them. There was also no bruising or tearing inside of my mouth, which is a big thing for me, as I always have problems with that during recovery. I also always have issues with the residual effects of general anesthesia, which are difficult, but with the sedation I was alert and responsive almost immediately after it was stopped. Best of all, there was no pain.

The whole staff at Dr. Fendrich's practice was wonderful, very coordinated, which made my recovery easier. I've already recommended having sedation dentistry done there to my cousin, who underwent chemotherapy that caused her to lose some teeth.

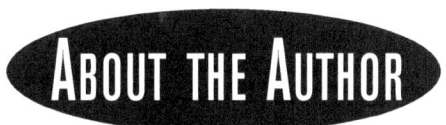

About the Author

Laurence E. Fendrich, DMD maintains offices in New York City and South Florida – concentrating on cosmetic and reconstructive dentistry, dental implants and IV sedation dentistry. He caters to a diverse group of people throughout the United States, Europe, the Caribbean and Central and South America. **Dr. Fendrich** is licensed as a general dentist and is IV moderate/conscious sedation certified in the states of New York and Florida.

▶ Dr. Fendrich

Is a graduate of Tufts University School of Dental Medicine and has been in practice for over thirty years. With a strong emphasis on cosmetic, reconstructive and implant dentistry, Dr. Fendrich has attended thousands of hours of continuing education to further his skills. He is a member of the American Dental Association, the Florida Dental Association, the New York State Dental Association and the American Dental Society of Anesthesiology.